POSTMODERN ENCOUNTERS

Donna Haraway and GM Foods

George Myerson

Series editor: Richard Appignanesi

ICON BOOKS UK

TOTEM BOOKS USA

Published in the UK in 2000
by Icon Books Ltd., Grange Road,
Duxford, Cambridge CB2 4QF
email: info@iconbooks.co.uk
www.iconbooks.co.uk

Published in the USA in 2001
by Totem Books
Inquiries to: Icon Books Ltd.,
Grange Road, Duxford,
Cambridge CB2 4QF, UK

Distributed in the UK, Europe,
Canada, South Africa and Asia
by the Penguin Group:
Penguin Books Ltd.,
27 Wrights Lane,
London W8 5TZ

In the United States,
distributed to the trade by
National Book Network Inc.,
4720 Boston Way, Lanham,
Maryland 20706

Library of Congress catalog
card number applied for

Published in Australia in 2001
by Allen & Unwin Pty. Ltd.,
PO Box 8500, 9 Atchison Street,
St. Leonards, NSW 2065

Text copyright © 2000 George Myerson

The author has asserted his moral rights.

Series editor: Richard Appignanesi

ISBN 1 84046 178 0

Typesetting by Wayzgoose

Printed and bound in the UK by
Cox & Wyman Ltd., Reading

For my daughter Elly, with love @
Second_Millennium.

The Strange Case of the Activist and the Monsters

Donna Haraway is a leading figure in contemporary feminist thought, and a major theorist of science and culture.[1] She is a declared activist, and ally of those who seek to resist exploitation, including the exploitation of the environment by big money and power. What would you *expect* her to think about genetically modified food? How would you *want* her to react? Surely she is an outspoken opponent of the new soya and corn, the alien fruits and vegetables? For these are beings, we hear, from Dr Frankenstein's Garden. Are the new engineered foodstuffs not another risk imposed on ordinary people by powerful companies? Is it not, then, the duty of all progressive thinkers to denounce the outrage committed on nature by greed?

Haraway herself sees that this expectation is natural. We like to know where our thinkers are coming from, just as much as we want to know where our food is coming from. She recognises that on 'the political left – my area of the political spectrum', the mood is unwelcoming to 'molecular genetics, biotechnology' and other such developments. Are these not just new means of 'profit and exploitation'?[2] Haraway is hardly a fan of Monsanto and the other gene genies, and she can feel the pull of her natural constituency, the radical activists and critics of established institutions. But she has a confession to make, and it is this confession which sets up a 'Postmodern Encounter':

I find myself especially drawn by such engaging new beings as the tomato with a gene from a cold-sea-bottom-living flounder . . .

How *could* she? And that's not the end of it! Haraway also has a weakness for 'the potato with a gene from a giant silk moth'.[3] Our encounter, then, will be between this influential feminist thinker and the monsters who have filled so many head-lines in the past few years.

The scene for the encounter is the book which Haraway published in 1997, with the weird title: *Modest_Witness@Second_Millennium. FemaleMan©_Meets_OncoMouse™*. It is in this book that she makes her confession, and her more general purpose is to respond to the new worlds which face us at the turn of the millennium. In addition to genetic foods, Haraway gazes upon all kinds of other new beings, virtual as well as biological, medical as well as theoretical. Her book is about the idea of a new era, at whose heart will be 'technoscience', the new hybrid of old sciences and technologies. What, she wants to know, should feminism make of the new dawn? How should any progressive critic of society respond to the changes, both actual and imminent, in the texture of everyday life and in the landscape of all our horizons?

As you can tell, it's a strange animal, this *Modest_Witness*. But there are three clear parts: in Part I, Haraway gives an account of technoscience; in Part II, she presents her 'meetings', between activist and fruit, between OncoMouse and FemaleMan, and between all kinds of other strange beings; and Part III offers a vista taking in 'gene' and 'fetus', 'race' and 'facts', in an overview of the prospects. Her encounter with the new fruits of the garden occurs in Part II, but its implications reverberate to and fro. *Modest_Witness* is not a book you can just read from beginning through to ending. It is full of echoes and linkages, repetitions and returns. There are academic footnotes and plenty of references to fellow scholars and experts. But the voice is fluid. One moment, we are reading a critique of an argument; then we move to a story, or a joke, or a personal recollection. In some ways, *Modest_Witness* is like a novel, and Haraway does draw as much upon fiction as upon academic sources. For example, she creates characters, or treats ideas as if they were characters. She herself becomes just one more character in her own world, along with other strangely-named presences, laboratory mice and FemaleMen. You can't extract a message from this kind of book, apart from the experience of reading it. So I have tried to re-create something of that experience, on the way to understanding 'The Strange Case of the Activist and the Monsters'. Why *does* Donna Haraway feel drawn to the moth-gened potato, or the flounder-spliced tomato?

Introducing an Alien

In May 1994, an alien being was sighted, by experts, making its way swiftly towards our familiar planet. This object, or creature, was heavily disguised, like all the best alien invaders, as something apparently harmless and familiar, something which we might walk past every day of our ordinary lives. Usually, aliens camouflage themselves as normal people, just like you and me, or like our neighbours. But this alien was even more devilishly cunning. After all, how many of us invite strangers right into our homes, however 'normal' they may be, or seem? No, that had been one of the flaws in previous alien plots. This time the aliens had a new plan. They no longer tried to pass themselves off as ordinary people. Instead, they were coming in the likeness of the humblest and most benign-looking objects. Yes, they had disguised themselves as vegetables! The cunning is almost beyond belief, even in retrospect, and the experts themselves, even the authorities, were very nearly deceived by it!

Like all the best invaders, the aliens were too crafty to land in a huge crowd. Instead, they had sent ahead one of their best spies, to try out the strategy. How close it came to working! For the master-stroke was that the alien had helpers already planted on the inside, or so one suspects in retrospect. Instead of arriving helpless and lonely, this alien being had its way carefully prepared in advance. On 18 May, messages began to appear to lull the public, and especially, of course, the American public, into a false sense of security. Associated Press (AP) spread across the continent a cryptic announcement of a coming 'vanguard' from a new and superior civilisation. On 19 May, AP adopted more ringing tones, declaring that this new being would be 'Coming Soon to a Store Near You'.

Suspiciously, with the wisdom of hindsight, all kinds of reassuring messages began being disseminated over the next few days. The AP of 19 May assured readers that they were about to receive benefits beyond those which old 'Mother Nature' had intended to bestow on them. Listen to the winning tones: this being will be 'attractive'; it is something we have 'often and strongly' desired; it has been certified as 'safe' by the highest authorities in the US. So the strategy began to take shape. Instead of sheltering behind the form of a familiar vegetable, keeping quiet and hoping to survive, this alien was carefully orchestrating the announcement of its imminent coming. It was a brilliant device, which almost paid off.

There was nothing secret about the landing of this alien vanguard. But in a way, this made the disguise all the more perfect. For, from every side, came voices declaring that we were about to meet a new 'US Tomato'.

Not only was the alien in the most harmless possible shape, but it was even a certified American being. This was the coming of the Flavr Savr, the 'Gene-Engineered US Tomato'. It was already on the inside, one of us, from the moment of its arrival. Indeed, it had voluntarily submitted to exhaustive tests by the US Food and Drugs authorities. Somewhere on its journey, this alien had even attracted terrestrial investment, to the tune of 20 million dollars!

Flavr Savr was a brilliant choice as the 'vanguard' of the alien vegetables and fruits. Just think about it: tomatoes are everywhere – in salads, of course, but especially in sauces and on pizzas, in pies and sandwiches. And everyone was fed up with the ordinary terrestrial varieties, which never had much taste when you got them from the supermarket, and which turned powdery on the tongue instead of staying crisp and juicy. Flavr Savr was also a great choice, because it was hardly an alien at all. It just had a little change or two in the ordinary genetic make-up of an earthly tomato.

As a biologist as well as a cultural critic, Donna Haraway is uniquely placed to spot the strategy. Some people claimed that this tomato was not really 'transgenic', not a true alien with a new and strange gene pattern. This was because it differed from the normal being only by having one gene reversed. This gene was meant to make the tomato ripen, and so rot, as expected. If the gene is reversed, the tomato stays fresh for longer. But Haraway spotted another change, the give-away. In her view, the new US tomato was 'strictly transgenic', because it had a gene added from a foreign source, a bacterium. This gene was used to keep track of the other changes, rather than to have any actual effect. Still, as Haraway says, it was no ordinary tomato: hidden within its code was an alien element, small and no doubt harmless as far as it goes, but as alien as they get.[4]

Bodies, Objects and Knowledge

The 'vanguard' tomato was subsequently withdrawn, and by now the association of 'genetic' with 'food' is not likely to figure large in anyone's advertising, certainly in Europe. Even in more friendly America, the biotechnology industry is on the defensive. There is something quite touching in retrospect about the article in *The Guardian* (21 May 1994) welcoming the tomato on behalf of Britain and Europe, with its reassurance about 'the astronomical number of genes we consume day by day'. Like the character in Molière who realises that he had always been talking prose, we have had to realise that we were always eating genes. Still, all food is genetic, but some foods are more genetic than others. The more recent controversies about genetically modified corn made clear, even to the biotech giant Monsanto, that the aliens had a long way to go before they would be seen as friends of the people. It seems that the issue has been wrapped up, and the aliens forced back into their spacecraft.

Let us follow Haraway, as she recalls that fateful moment in May 1994, to see why this is unlikely to be the end of the story. Part II of *Modest_Witness* gives an account of modern science. In the 19th century, as she tells it, chemistry brought order to the inorganic world through the Periodic Table of Elements. This table led scientists to predict the presence of various elements before they were discovered, including uranium. Then science added to the table of naturally occurring elements, the fateful additions including plutonium and other 'transuranic elements'. Meanwhile, evolutionary theory and genetics were bringing an equal order to the biological realm. Human beings belong to both of these systems.

Then Haraway interrupts her own story: 'On the day I wrote the preceding paragraph, May 19th 1994, front pages of newspapers all over the United States reported that the U.S. Food and Drugs Administration had given its final approval to Calgene, Inc. . . . to put its genetically-

engineered tomato, the Flavr Savr, on the market.'
She puts 19 May 1994 up there in lights, as a red-
letter day in the history of science and society.
True, there is a touch of mockery. But amidst the
ambiguity, she goes on to explain why the tomato
is so significant. Flavr Savr 'does not decay as
fast' as its natural counterparts. This engineered
slow-down in the rate of decay makes an exact
analogy between the 'transgenic' tomato and the
'transuranic' element, plutonium, whose length-
ened half-life is so much a part of the dangerous
history of nuclear power.[5]

Haraway puts the vanguard tomato alongside
the radioactive powerhouse, plutonium, as two
of the trinity of 'key synthetic objects' that have
defined the phases of 'the last century of the
Second Christian Millennium: nylon, plutonium,
and transgenics'.[6] These are no mere objects, they
are also 'revolutionary new world citizens'. These
are entities in whose presence the entire world is
altered. The texture and fabric of everyday life
shifts in the face of these beings, and history is
never the same again. These are new types of
object. Their successive appearance revises what

it means to be an object at all. They redraw the boundaries of the object on earth. Nylon comes to us from 'synthetic organic chemistry', plutonium from 'transuranic nuclear generation', and lastly we have the contribution of 'genetic engineering'. The claim could not be clearer. The world can no more spring back into place after the appearance in our midst of Flavr Savr than it could after the invention of plutonium or of nylon.

But here, precisely, is the ambiguity: is the new genetic object going to be another plutonium or another nylon? Is this new wave of alien objects going to be the fatal invasion or a benign enriching? Haraway isn't telling: she doesn't want to give answers. Her aim, instead, is to bring before our eyes the deep ambiguity of the moment which surfaced with Flavr Savr: 'Transgenic organisms are at once completely ordinary and the stuff of science fiction.' If you look clearly at these objects, you lose all your certainties, and you find yourself facing a horizon of questions. These new things are embodiments of the next 'world-shaping' science: they will be to biology what plutonium was to physics and nylon to chemistry.[7]

Modest_Witness wants us to have a language with which to discuss these new beings and our new experiences and feelings in their presence. Haraway returns us repeatedly to her keyword 'transgenic', and defines for us any 'transgenic organism' as one which has genes 'transplanted' across biological boundaries, between species or even biological kingdoms, such as plant and animal. In her sentences, there is always a flash of humorous wonder at having to share the world with such entities at last, beings in whom genes have passed 'from fish to tomatoes, fireflies to tobacco, bacteria to humans'.[8] For the present, 'food crops' are the field where the genes are at their liveliest and most mobile: but other beings are not far behind. Haraway declares that these entities redefine the whole system of 'kinship relations' within which we live.[9] Where once there were clear divisions, now there are questionable connections. Tomatoes can inherit a little from fish, with a helping hand. Flavr Savr is not just a different object from the conventional tomato: it belongs to a different world, where other possibilities exist. In that sense, the alien invasion has already been carried

17

out. Nothing is the same, already. All food was always genetic, but not in the way it is now.

Haraway has given her book an e-mail address rather than a conventional title: another kind of new label, for a new world, perhaps. She is making a link between several new worlds. One is the genetic world of Flavr Savr and also other beings such as OncoMouse, whom we shall soon meet. Another is the cultural world where 'FemaleMan' originates, as a character in a novel and also as a sign that old categories are cracking. But let us pause on that '@' and visit a website, www.monsanto.co.uk. This is the home site of the main biotech company in the agricultural area, and here we find a helpful 'Biotech Primer' of human history. Here, too, 1994 is a crucial date.

1994. First authorisation by the EU to market a transgenic plant: a tobacco plant.
First commercialisation of a transgenic plant in the United States: delayed ripening tomato . . .

Looking forward, we arrive at . . .

1996. The European Union approved the importation and use of Monsanto's Roundup Ready Soya bean . . .

But now just see what happens when you look back:

Tens of Thousands of years ago. People wandered the earth, collecting and eating only what they found growing in nature.

In between this poor world of nature, and the future, come the stages of agriculture and then the rise of genetics. Confronted by this 'timeline', it is easy to recoil and spring to the defence of poor old 'nature', viewing those soybeans as another advance party in the alien invasion of the genetic foods. No one has given a more dramatic warning than Haraway herself, when she offers the parallel between those two synthetic objects, transgenic organisms like Flavr Savr and transuranic elements like plutonium. But equally, she cannot repress a touch of 'curiosity and frank pleasure in the recent doings of flounders and tomatoes'. Not all new worlds are brave new worlds; let us look again at the alien vanguard.

Cyborgs, Tomatoes and Rats

In Haraway's terms, the new synthetic organisms are part of the wider world of 'cyborgs'. She is a long-time student of 'cyborg figures'. Though, as she acknowledges, Haraway did not invent the term 'cyborg', she has been the most important developer of the concept, and it provides her with another way of thinking about the invading tomato and the unfamiliar soybeans. In sci-fi terms, cyborgs are hybrids in which, particularly, organic and cybernetic, or synthetic, elements are mixed. So you might say that an obvious example would be someone with a pacemaker implanted. But Haraway largely sweeps aside such obvious instances. She has bigger fish to fry, and is not interested in the cyborg exception, but in the rule of the cyborgs. She states firmly that, for her, cyborgs are 'not about the Machine and the Human', because she does not see these categories as fixed or stable. There are not fixed humans, any more than there are fixed tomatoes or, for that matter, fixed computers. All these entities are changing, under various influences, all the time. Cyborgs are beings in whose presence the categories themselves break down. A flounder-gened tomato does not leave untouched the categories of plant and animal, or fish and fruit, or natural and man-made. In its extra-fresh presence, we can no longer talk with confidence of these categories at all.

For Haraway, the genetic engineering story is all about this break-down of categories. She sees one of her own main functions as being to challenge the accepted definitions and divisions, particularly, as a feminist, the divisions of the world by gender. Therefore, she has a professional, as well as a personal, attachment to 'my cyborg figures'. Their upsurge into the world announces the bending of all the old concepts. Furthermore, the cyborgs are themselves fellow-inhabitants of some of our own new worlds. They share with us the new patterns of 'technobiopower', which is bending the very time and space in which we all dwell. Time speeds up, in some places, under this new regime: things grow faster, messages move more quickly. But elsewhere time has been slowing down: tomatoes decay more patiently, just as plutonium did before them. Time is simply not what it was – time is changing.

Our old familiar time bends and wobbles in the presence of such objects as Flavr Savr. Haraway gazes across the ranks of other time-warping presences in our new lives: 'Cyborg figures – such as the end-of-the-millennium seed, chip, gene, database, bomb, fetus, race, brain, and ecosystem . . .'[10] Each of these figures has the weird property of re-routing time and space. The new 'seed', like Monsanto's genetically-engineered soybean, grows according to many new laws: more quickly, more enduringly, in new places. The 'gene' has redefined for us the meaning of the future, and therefore of the present in its turn. The future is coming closer: its presence is ready-to-hand for us. The new 'fetus' is increasingly following rhythms of our dictation, and we are more and more able to read its secrets, perhaps even to re-write them. The new 'bomb' is smart, like us. The 'ecosystem' is a being that has arisen as we have become conscious of destroying it: it is the presence of a threatened future. The 'database' is a new entity, a being composed of information – in the image of the gene.

Genetically-engineered food is itself the offspring of several of these cyborg figures: seed, gene, database. It is thus close kin to other such offspring, among whom Haraway picks out particularly a small rodent, OncoMouse, a lab mouse genetically redesigned to grow cancers. It is thus a customised tool for cancer research and, as Haraway points out, it may be our saviour: in its suffering may lie our hope of deliverance. OncoMouse is as time-altering as Flavr Savr or plutonium. Its future pain is as tightly coded as Flavr Savr's refusal to rot. In the presence of these beings, categories melt: present and future, chance and fate, nature and culture. We made them, and we now inhabit the new time-and-space which they have brought into being around them.

Like Flavr Savr, OncoMouse is a first. It has its own patent, held by Harvard University, with the commercial rights held by DuPont. In the presence of OncoMouse, we cannot apply as we used to the categories of law and nature. As Haraway says, OncoMouse has for its 'natural habitat' the lab and its social setting – from the Corporation which sells it, to the State which made the rules and gave the cash. In the old alien romances, the problem was to tell when you were in the presence of an alien. They gave off strange vibrations, to which some people were fortunately sensitive. You can tell you are in the presence of a cyborg figure when you feel a new world coming into being around you. In the case of OncoMouse, this is 'the world of corporate biology', a world that reaches from the gene to the corporate share, from the breeding centre to the hospital. We share the future with OncoMouse: the prospects of cancer and the possibilities of cure.

When OncoMouse appeared, the request for a patent was opposed by animal rights groups who argued that this was a travesty of life, a being designed to suffer. Scientists replied that this suffering was our best hope for relief, ours and our children's. *Modest_Witness* is not the kind of place to go for answers. It is a book of strange worlds, new connections. Cyborg ethics sees clearly that both sides are inevitable accompaniments of OncoMouse's birth. These responses are part of the meaning of this creature. Haraway reaches towards a new kind of ethics, a different commitment. She derives from a novel by Joanna Russ the figure of the FemaleMan©, in whom the old categories of gender are as redundant as the old nature and culture are in OncoMouse™. Haraway then declares, on behalf of FemaleMan, the meeting of the hybrids, the time-warpers, the victim-champions of the new age: 'OncoMouse is my sibling, male or female, s/he is my sister.'[11]

As you can tell, Haraway's book is itself a cyborg: research report and confession, history and prophecy, academic analysis and poetic fiction. Her business is neither to denounce nor to endorse the new beings. But neither is she merely reporting. She aims to share the world with Flavr Savr and OncoMouse. Hers is the reverse of the old alien story – it is all about recognising the new family, the extended family into which we have been re-born as cyborg citizens. The era of the nuclear family may be passing; the transgenic family is on the way, with its new sibling rivalries and affections.

www.hypercapitalism.com

SEVEN MORE GENETICALLY ENGINEERED FOODS ARE SAFE

Now the agency* has completed . . . inspections of seven other genetically altered plants . . .

– Three more tomatoes . . .

– A squash genetically altered to naturally resist two deadly viruses . . .

– A potato that naturally resists the Colorado potato beetle . . .

*US Food and Drugs Administration

AP, 2/11/1994

Capitalism manufactured objects, and in doing so it also manufactured a world, and the lives within it. Now something different is happening to the objects, and so, it follows, capitalism has taken a new turning. New objects are cascading among us. Only a few months after Flavr Savr, and here come the super-tomatoes, the resistant squash and the new potato. The key word in this announcement is 'naturally'. In what sense do these beings 'naturally' exist at all, let alone possess the new powers advertised? These things are neither natural nor unnatural, in the old senses: they are beyond natural and unnatural. That is why, in Haraway's terms, 'The offspring of these technoscientific wombs are cyborgs . . .'. What we have here is no longer the mass manufacture of objects that belong to us and not to nature. Instead, we have the beginnings of a new organic regime, blessed with unimaginable fertility, giving birth to infinite possibilities, all of them in their own way 'natural'. Instead of manufacturing objects, we are re-creating the process of birth. This is a new nature, rather than a non-nature or an anti-nature.

Haraway adds that these cyborgs carry within themselves 'densely packed condensations of worlds'. In that potato, for example, there is the potential world where the old plagues are harmless; what was lethal is now mundane. The Colorado beetle will become a symbol of a vanished order, if that world comes into full being. The squash may realise a world where viruses are innocuous, the 'deadly' agents defused for ever. Clearly these possibilities reach well beyond potato blight and squash rot: we are looking out towards the horizon where other plagues and deadly agents are harmless.

Bill Gates and Paul Allen, the billionaire co-founders of Microsoft, have invested $10 million in a new biopharmaceutical company. The company, Seattle-based Darwin Molecular Corp., said it plans to develop treatments for AIDS, cancer and autoimmune diseases through computer analysis of DNA.

The Washington Post, 7/5/1994

You can see why Haraway has given her genetic vision an e-mail address. DNA becomes another network on the world wide web of information. The new company, Darwin Molecular, will itself be a cyborg, a hybrid in whose presence neither DNA nor IT will have their old meaning. And spinning the web are 'the billionaire co-founders of Microsoft' by whose courtesy indeed this text is being written. Both OncoMouse and Flavr Savr will be perfectly at home in this network of connected worlds, where life and information have undergone a mega-merger to form the biggest corporation of all.

' . . . for AIDS, cancer and autoimmune diseases': another cascade tumbles down towards us, a cascade of info-beings which will cure everything. Without these diseases, health and well-being will join the long list of redundant categories. Being healthy will have either no meaning, or a new meaning, in a world where the old scourges have been defused. Our bodies, like the other objects, will have escaped the old categories through which we have viewed them. Darwin Molecular, like the gene and the ecosystem, is a cyborg packed with worlds waiting to be born.

Across the financial pages, and among our lives, floods an ever-accelerating torrent of new beings. Haraway calls the procession 'hypercapitalist market traffic', and at times the volume of traffic threatens gridlock. Capitalism has gone hyper: faster, weirder, more extravagant, more fictional. This is the real traffic problem facing the new millennium. Hypercapitalism leaves nothing untransformed in its pursuit of growth and profitability. All objects suddenly have the potential to transform without giving us any notice. Tomatoes, rats, human bodies, viruses, cells, databases: objects join hands, they meet, greet and dance together, to the tune of hyper-capitalism.

But the earth itself is just another object from this point of view. Why should this object be any different? According to Haraway, in tune with the social theory of Beck, Giddens and Castells, the old earth is passing away, and a new earth is being born. We are witnessing the 'globalisation of the world'. Flavr Savr has been adapted to surpass every local idiosyncrasy; similarly, OncoMouse is on a universal quest. These beings address the whole earth: they are made for that purpose. As the net spreads across, as the old earth becomes the new global system, the hybrid age arrives – the age of which the tomato and the lab rat are symbols, prophets and perhaps fellow-victims.

The market for life is a volatile place. Every being is potentially connected to all the others, and each new link makes its world afresh. Standing further back, Haraway places this global planet in a new 'technoscientific planetary space', orbited not by the moon so much as by com-munications satellites. If you want to understand what this new planet is like, your best bet is by 'tracing radioisotopes through food chains'.[12] Then you will see just how intricate are the interconnecting networks into which these new entities have fallen. No wonder the financial news of the day is all about mergers. Indeed, to adapt Haraway, just a week before I wrote these words, Time Warner and AOL merged to create the biggest cyborg of them all, the old-new media-Internet company, the traditional avant-garde hybrid, the geek-gened film company, the film-gened book publisher. (Then, as I returned to the text, they both merged with EMI; things have speeded up even since 1994, it seems.)

Inserting a bacterium gene into a tomato is one small change in vegetable marketing; but it is also one large change in the international economy. Flavr Savr and OncoMouse are among the first fully naturalised citizens of the new global earth. They are the rightful inhabitants of 'transnational enterprise culture', which Haraway labels 'the New World Order, Inc'. Nuclear physics was the patron science of the Cold War world; trans-genics is the science of this New World Order.[13]

Impurity Hall

Haraway is not celebrating the onset of hyper-capitalism. On the contrary, she sees power moving ever further away from the places where most people live. Yet she feels sympathy, even empathy, for the new beings that are born in the wombs of technoscience. The most moving aspect of *Modest_Witness@Second_Millennium* is the affirmation of kinship with all the other non-standard beings. Therefore, if you look through Haraway's eyes, or those of her characters, like OncoMouse and FemaleMan, you will have mixed feelings when you read of Flavr Savr's fate:

. . . activists from his Pure Food Campaign would protest the tomato . . .

The Washington Post, 21/5/1994

Haraway repeatedly calls herself an 'activist', and she is intuitively sympathetic to all campaigners against the global powers. Yet her work also suggests a reservation about any demand for a return to lost purity. Is Flavr Savr bad because it is impure, her hybrid voices lead one to ask?

This is the troubled heart of the encounter between Donna Haraway and genetic foods, this question of purity and impurity:

GM CROPS: GENETIC POLLUTION PROVED

Friends of the Earth Press Release,
www.foe.org.uk, 10.30 p.m., 29/9/1999

The immediate concern was field trials of GM corn, and the 'genetic pollution' referred to the spread of alien pollen. But the phrase 'genetic pollution' also has its other lives, its deeper resonances, whatever the good intentions of those using it. Elsewhere, the Soil Association, voice of organic farming, opposed the same trials on the grounds of 'cross-contamination' (Briefing Paper, June 1999, www.Soilassociation.org), and defended the destruction of GM trial crops; Lord Melchett of Greenpeace referred to 'decontamination'. On the other wing of the argument, we find the 'bio-engineers':

BIO-ENGINEERS FIND A WAY TO 'CONTAIN' SUPER PLANTS

Researchers at Auburn University have developed a technique that they say should wilt fears that genetically altered plants will spread their genes around.

www.CNN.com, 23/4/1998

The dominant voices of *Modest_Witness* are more attuned to Greenpeace than to Monsanto, and indeed Haraway is sharply ironic at the expense of a Monsanto-sponsored biology textbook, seeing in it a crude justification of a vested interest, disguised as science education. And yet, while recognising the terrifying forces at work in hypercapitalism, Haraway recoils at the heart of the anti-genetic food arguments, at just that point where, probably, the arguments have been most persuasive and influential.

In most protests, the new genetically-modified food, and food crops, appear to be impurities. They are illegitimate hybrids. Phrases like 'genetic pollution' inevitably come to life in these arguments. The problem isn't the intentions of the campaigners or the immediate thrust of the campaigns. The problem is that this kind of language is haunted. There are ghosts, and perhaps demons, in the metaphors of endangered purity and genetic contamination. These spirits pay no heed to the aims or meanings of the campaigners – they are just riding back to life within the words.

Modest_Witness is always seeking out the viewpoint of the hybrid, the illicit, the uncategorised being. From that kind of viewpoint, you hear at work, in the most admirable campaigns, the old Western demons 'obsessed with racial purity'. Here is the most difficult act of witnessing. In the name of all the aliens, the unclean, the uncategorised of the world, Haraway commits all her many voices to an act of commemoration:

It is a mistake in this context to forget that anxiety over the pollution of lineages is at the origin of racist discourse in European cultures.

Haraway is always intuitively with the activists. Her argument isn't that they are unconsciously racist. But in the language there live the ghosts of other voices, the demons of the old and undead racism of the ages. From the perspective of the cyborgs, the hybrids, such language as 'genetic pollution' can never be innocent of its past, and always risks appealing to the same old reactions, however benign and progressive the immediate intentions.

I cannot help but hear in the biotechnology debates the unintended tones of fear of the alien and suspicion of the mixed.

Haraway's argument is uncompromising, and everything in the book – the way it is written as much as its message – contributes to this moment. You cannot exploit the logic of natural 'kind and purity' at the end of the second millennium without setting foot on haunted ground.

As far as genetics and food goes, then, *Modest_Witness@Second_Millennium* has a mixed message. This technology is inseparable from hypercapitalism, with its global reach and ambition. But biotechnology is also not identical with this economic system; there is more at work than mere instrumental exploitation. In particular, Haraway wants us to recoil from some of the most influential arguments against genetically modified foods, and crops, and organisms. If you are going to argue against, then you will need to look elsewhere than 'the doctrine of types and intrinsic purposes'. There never was a nature in which all the categories were pure; and it can never be an intrinsic argument against a phenomenon that it involves 'border-crossing' or transgressing categories. If there are things wrong with the new beings, and their sponsors, then it's not their mixed nature that is at fault. Can you really (asks the voice of the witness) believe that, after the 20th century, good will come of arguing against 'implanted alien genes'? Is it really going to be possible to limit the influence of these metaphors to the field in which they are being planted?[14]

Haraway recalls that in 1938, when DuPont first began the commercial manufacture of nylon, the work was based at a new lab called Purity Hall. It seems, one might elaborate, that the new science of transgenics will be better based at 'Impurity Hall'. This science will breed beings whom others may denounce as 'disharmonious crosses'; it will revel in 'alien genes', which will seem threatening to those who imagine the world used to be pure. Impurity Hall will be as much a centre of capitalism, gone hyper, as Purity Hall was for the earlier phase. This is not a place from which liberation, in any simple sense, will flow among the nations of the world.

Yet there is a positive potential to the science, whatever the dangers involved in its exploitation and ownership. This new 'technoscience' itself will always be a hybrid of pure and applied, commercial and arcane, practice and theory. As the new biology goes about its business of extracting profits, it will also be the agent that 'mixes up all the actors'. In the wake of biological technoscience, the pseudo-scientific basis of 'racial purity' will at last fall into final disrepute. The world will reveal itself, irreversibly, as a place of burgeoning ambiguities. The cause of pure categories may at last be defeated, and the victorious heroes will include 'a bastard mouse', all the cross-patched humans who are its kith and kin, and their endlessly mixed progeny.[15]

Do you feel the world turning upside-down, dear reader? Remember, this supposedly *Modest Witness* is a dangerous character, one who feels drawn to the aliens. Isn't the argument usually the other way round – that the new genetics has sinister links with the old so-called sciences of population control and manipulation, once known as 'eugenics'? Is it not the genetic manipulators who belong to the camp of the race purifiers? Do they not keep alive old dreams of rooting out 'degenerates' by genetic reprogramming? *Modest Witness* testifies against that claim: s/he finds, in the transgenic creatures, allies of all that is unsound, hybrid, anomalous, and, s/he adds, lively and full of the diversity of surprising futures.

Let us have a closer look at this witness . . .

Mutating the Modest Witness

Scientific ideas have always created controversy, both within and beyond science. Nevertheless, looking back as Haraway is doing over the second millennium, science has been a pretty successful way of achieving 'credible witness' in a world where people are bound to disagree about everything they touch. Considering how well-programmed we are to take issue with one another, science has often possessed a truly 'stunning power', none other than the ability 'to establish matters of fact' on many issues, as far as many of its contemporaries have been concerned. In religion and in politics, disagreement rules, and the facts are perpetually in doubt. Facts fuel the arguments between politicians, religious leaders and moral factions. Just listen to a news debate. One side claims that the facts show the economy is improving, and then a torrent of alternative facts pours down on the other side. We find this natural: it is our home, this arguable world. Yet science has been different for the last centuries of the millennium. In those societies where science has become established, people have got used to accepting *scientific* facts as different from ordinary facts. Of course, there is always room to argue about what counts as a science, and there is never a shortage of dissident scientists. But an amazing array of facts has been kept like islands in the rolling oceans of our disputes. These have been facts about all kinds of subjects that we could not possibly check or even question. We have adopted facts about the birth of the universe, or the nature of matter, facts about the origin of species or the development of humanity, facts about the nervous system or the nature of sound.

Science has made facts *believable* in a world of arguments. Haraway tells the story by creating a character called the 'modest witness'. This witness speaks with the scientific voice, and, in the right court, he (for it has been a 'he', predominantly) will be believed, if he issues statements about fact. Haraway is entranced by this lucid authority. The modest witness has seemed to be speaking on behalf of 'the object world'. Everyone else is subjective, and what they say derives from their point of view. But the modest witness is the exception. In his words, we hear the objects speaking, whether they are stones or neurones. The modest witness has been able to ensure 'the clarity and purity of objects'. Thanks to this voice, we know what things are and what they are not.[16]

The new technoscience is different. It challenges the purity of objects. After Flavr Savr, 'tomato' is an ambiguous category, and withdrawing the brand will not alter the effect. The point, of course, is that things always were ambiguous – they overlapped behind our backs, they put out links and held hands when we weren't looking. We have just begun to wake up to the many alliances. Nature no longer stands for purity. But in what voice, then, shall these objects be witnessed? Clearly, the old modest witness will not speak on their behalf.

Take the case of the monarch butterfly. In 1999, research at Cornell University suggested that pollen from modified corn was toxic to the caterpillars of the much-loved monarch butterfly. Friends of the Earth drew this to the attention of President Clinton:

. . . the alarming new study by scientists at Cornell University . . . find(s) that nearly half of the monarch caterpillars feeding on Bt. corn pollen died after four days . . .

www.foe.org, 14/6/1999

Of course, facts have always been disputed, even when 'scientists' announced them. But there is something different about these disputes. In Britain, Prince Charles asks whether we really understand these monster crops. In reply, Professor Dereck Burke acerbically comments that:

The well publicised experiments with the Monarch butterfly show that under laboratory conditions caterpillars force-fed corn pollen are damaged . . .

Feedback Magazine, 14/6/1999

There is no distance here between 'the science' and 'the media'. The scientific witness has lost its independence from politics, or religion, where genetic modification is in dispute. No one sees the scientist as an independent witness here; indeed, that is not what this science is for. Here, science has become a dimension of controversy. These claims do not begin as neutral science and then become embroiled in the contentions of politics and religion and ethics. No, these are the claims by which science stirs up the controversies in the first place. In this new world, science and controversy have been spliced as surely as the flounder and the tomato.

But then, where does the book itself speak from? Haraway commits her book early on to a 'contaminated practice'.[17] It would not make sense for *Modest_Witness@Second_Millennium* to speak objectively about the passing of pure objectivity, or neutrally about the obsolescence of scientific neutrality. Haraway's book speaks from an address within the world it interprets. Since that world is impure everywhere you turn, the text can hardly be an island of purity. What is the 'contamination'? In the debates about modified pollen, campaigners refer to the 'contamination' of the environment by alien genes. Haraway's words accept their own contamination. They are nowhere pure. For example, this is a work of social science, drawing upon literatures in anthropology, cultural studies and sociology of science. But it is also a work of fiction, in its format, style and, most important, its thinking. The sentences start out as propositions, turn into metaphorical visions and then uncoil again to yield arguments.

The old-style modest witness aimed to persuade by being, or seeming, transparent. 'These are just the facts; they speak for themselves.' But Haraway is not dealing with a world where such facts occur frequently. They are at least an endangered species. Facts have become contentious claims in arguments in which the status of the parties is precisely the issue. Who does speak for science, anyway?

Haraway's text doesn't just talk about ideas. The words actually seem to come *from* the ideas, they seem able to speak for themselves. For example, Haraway gives an objective-seeming account of OncoMouse, 'the finely-tailored laboratory rodents'. But soon she turns the picture inside-out, declaring that the rodent's 'mutated murine eyes' are the source of her point of view. This text aims to place its sentences inside the perspectives of the ideas and beings it is analysing. These are the moments of affirmation: 'I adopt FemaleMan as my surrogate . . .' Both Female-Man and OncoMouse live 'after the implosion' in which objectivity and subjectivity, fact and metaphor, collapsed into each other. Haraway is not saying that there are not facts. On the contrary: the book is full of statements which are false if they aren't true, information about biology, about population, about disease and health. But there are not 'pure' facts here; they bring with them contention, they are always within the field of a dispute. If there were no dispute, no one would bother to collect this information and claim it as a fact.

Our guiding text is made in the image of the creatures it is interpreting: the moth-proofed potato, the cancer-prone rat, the super-squash. Would you trust a guide to such a weird world if s/he sounded familiar and straightforward? There are moments when the author, or her voice, seems to be taken over by the world. Looking inwards, Haraway the writer finds strange births happening in her own words: 'Narrative timescapes proliferate in the flesh of my sentences . . . '; the past is spliced to the future, the story of progress to the parable of disaster.[18]

The crucial question is this: who are we to trust in the new world? This question reaches far beyond genetic food to a host of environmental issues, health crises and risks. We are in a phase where *trust* itself is the main subject at issue. The disputes about genetic food are strong examples of this more general trend. The problem is to decide what kind of voice to believe. Haraway is not telling you what to believe. But she is suggesting that you re-think what kind of witness you trust.

The FemaleMan and OncoMouse are, finally, modest witnesses to world-changing matters of fact . . .

You had better start trusting the ambiguous ones, the voices which cannot be defined. If you want to understand these new facts, then try imagining them from the perspective of the cancer-prone saviour rat. Seek out the most ambiguous viewpoint, and re-view the facts from there. In effect, Haraway is claiming that the new genetic facts are not just more information. They represent a change in the whole nature of information. Facts are not what they used to be. These ideas, of course, are themselves ambiguous! But one of the things they mean is that these facts are spliced with all kinds of uncertainties. These are not facts that are cut-

and-dried. They include possibilities, a whole calculus of what might and might not happen.

Let's recall Flavr Savr, and GM corn, and moth potato. Put the question to them: are you safe? The answer takes the form of statements about probability, including the probabilities of harm from other foods, like 'normal' burgers or chips or chocolate. In addition, the facts about genetic foods are saturated facts; they are suffused by theories. You can't separate the basic information about Flavr Savr from complex theories about DNA or about evolution itself. Haraway calls such data 'world-changing matters of fact': these are facts within certain worlds.[19] In other words, to accept the 'fact' that a squash is now 'naturally' resistant to decay involves entering a certain world, and leaving another one behind. In that new world, there are new facts. But if you stay in the old world, these will not look like the 'facts'. This doesn't mean that someone isn't right, someone else wrong. But it means that we will need new ways of deciding.

Haraway is writing with a purpose, call it even a moral purpose, in the sense that novelists can have a moral purpose: 'I want a mutated modest witness . . .' The old modest witnesses were plausible experts. They spoke objectively about experiments which yielded clear results. They referred their arguments to scientific theories which were accepted by strong expert communities. Somewhere at the end of the second millennium, we stopped trusting those old witnesses. The cynical explanation is that they gave one too many reassurances that turned out false, or warnings that turned out unnecessary. We gave up butter, only to find ourselves recommended it again. We were told that British beef was safe to eat, and then the roof fell in. But Haraway has a deeper explanation. The facts have become more complicated. They have changed their nature. A fact about Flavr Savr is just not the same kind of thing as a fact about oak trees, or rubber, or the moon. It has more in common with facts about, say, Black Holes, or programming 'languages'. These are 'mutated' facts – full of theories, full of uncertainties and ambiguities. You have to grasp these new facts as much with your imagination as with your calculator.

49

Mutant Universities

A scientific article about genes and food is a form of knowledge, or would-be knowledge; so, in a different way, is a newspaper article. But the Flavr Savr is also a form of knowledge, and not just any other being in the world. Similarly, a book about cancer aims to be accepted as knowledge. A news item aims to spread, or question, that knowledge. But OncoMouse is also a form of knowledge, as well as a means of gaining further information. Knowledge can take the form of words, or of objects, and even, now, of living beings.

Universities try to produce knowledge, much of it in the form of texts. But they also produce the new living knowledge, the information-organisms. Let us summon OncoMouse again, this time to bear witness to the nature of her creator.

MUTANT MICE IN EUROPEAN TEST CASE
Mutant mice bred by Harvard University turned into a test case . . .

AP, 21/1/1993

This item is about the European legal battle to secure a patent for OncoMouse for its original inventors, Harvard University. The university, as we have seen, already held the patent in the US:

Its US patent was granted in 1988, the first ever for an artificially engineered natural life form.

The creature seems to be alarming because it breaks all the boundaries: artificial and natural, engineered and living. But the news report also emphasises that its ownership is equally hybrid:

DuPont de Nemours and Bio, Inc. of Wilmington, Delaware own the commercial rights.

The mouse is an academic product and a commercial commodity; it is a research tool and a space in a sales catalogue; it is the hope of a cure and the gleam of a profit. All the categories are in flux together, and among them is the university itself. In making OncoMouse, Harvard also remade itself. OncoMouse, by its presence, testifies to something fundamental about Harvard and its kin: they too have a new family system.

If knowledge is changing, then you would expect the institutions of learning and research to change too. Harvard is spliced with DuPont, the company we saw earlier at the heart of the plastics revolution and then the atomic age. This splicing is the inevitable complement to the new genetic inventions. Spliced institutions create the hybrid world within which such inventions occur. OncoMouse's natural habitat is this place where Harvard and DuPont merge. Other genetic innovations will inhabit an even more ambiguous world:

The Cambridge Massachusetts-based Millennium researchers, collaborating with Switzerland-based Hoffman-La Roche as well as other pharmaceutical labs and academic centers, have been seeking the receptor gene . . .

AP, 29/12/1995

You can no longer say where the academic centres stop and the commercial organisations start;

nor can you be sure where the USA stops and Switzerland starts. More subtly, you can't be sure where pharmaceutics stops and genetics starts. The university used to be a system of well-patrolled borders – between disciplines, and between the academy and various outside worlds. True, there were many secret crossings; but now that there is a new age, the border controls have been removed. Instead, from these 'academic centres' flies a flag with the motto: Welcome to the hybrid world!

In the previous section, we saw Haraway exploring the ambiguities of her own writing, and of communication in general. She is equally interested in these institutions, or networks, where knowledge is created. She traces, for example, the inter-linkage of Harvard and DuPont back to the late 1970s in the biotech field, and sees the connection as 'a trademark of the symbiosis between industry and academia'.[20] Trademarks belong to the economic world; symbiosis is part of nature. Again, the categories curve into each other. So, again, the 'basic technique of gene splicing' is covered by a spliced patent, the Stanley-Cohen-Herbert-Boyer Patent. The ownership passes across two universities, Stanford and the University of California at San Francisco, and there are added industrial interests. Haraway is trying to show the logic of a world in action. Here, nothing stays distinct and separate. To exist is to have a potential for becoming connected to other entities, for being absorbed or overlapped or redefined. The university is no different from the tomato in this respect: it has no clear boundaries, but exists in relation with other entities. There is no firm inside and outside to the university, any more than there is to the squash.

Haraway can see only too clearly how these overlaps and mergers could look like another kind of corruption. Are we not losing our institutes of 'pure' learning? Kin of OncoMouse, admirer of deviant flounders, Haraway has no time for this melancholy. She denounces 'nostalgia for "pure research"' on several grounds. For one thing, knowledge never was pure, it only tried to appear pure. For another thing, the hybrid mentality is fundamentally creative. She refers, for example, to 'the complex splice between computer science and molecular biology', a splice out of which the new genetics has evolved. True, there is plenty to worry about in the 'corporatization of biology', which is a less happy way to describe the 'symbiosis' of university and industry. The serious danger is the threat to 'social criticism'. Will universities that depend on these huge partnerships still be home to critics of the same economic system? It is not purity that is the loss, but criticism, itself a mixed-up hybrid activity, part intellect and part emotion, part detachment and part involvement.[21]

The book's address specifies a time: *@Second_Millennium*. The turn of the millennium is itself a hybrid time, where eras are spliced together, and where memory and prophecy intermingle. In that moment, the university also mutates, and Haraway with it, for she is writing from one such mutant. With shades of disgust, of anger and of hope, she seeks to bear witness within this changed institution, and that is one of the main reasons why she has taken so much care over the genetic new wave. For these product-

beings carry within themselves the pattern of our institutes of learning: spliced, incongruous and potentially creative. We tend to think of knowledge as being part of the search to discover the truth about our world. But for Haraway the new knowledge is made of 'world-making practices'. That is, knowledge now seizes upon the world and re-makes it. In the 18th century, the first botanical scientists classified the plants; at the turn of the millennium, their hybrid descendants are re-mixing the categories. You could say new connections are being revealed, or that new links are being made, or that the true boundaries are being destroyed. Is nature yielding her true secrets, when the flounder comes to the rescue of the decaying tomato? In Haraway's terms, the answer is 'yes and no': we are helping to reshape nature, from within, at the same time as we seek understanding.

Haraway adopts the principle that 'Nothing comes without its world'. In the case of Flavr Savr, or genetically modified soybean, that world includes the mutant universities of the second millennium. Does the world create these beings, or do they create that world? There is no clear answer. Without the new world, there are no new beings, and without the new beings, there is no new world. Haraway talks, ambiguously, of 'forging knowledges': who can say any longer exactly when knowledge is genuine? Throughout the Cold War, social theorists talked of the 'military-industrial complex'. Now, Haraway suggests, we can also talk of the academic-industrial complex, a huge system that forges new knowledge in hundreds of brilliant new ways. We live in the age of the knowledge forgers, and they are the ones who have sent as their 'vanguard' Flavr Savr and GM corn and OncoMouse.[22]

The Transgenic Millennium

We began with the question of whether the world would soon be seeing the last of the genetic foods. Haraway explains why these beings are not going to leave us alone. The vegetable mutants aren't going to get back into their space capsules and head for home. The reason isn't so much to do with the economics of food marketing, or consumer demand, or the supermarket retail system, or attitudes towards health and risk. All of those factors have a short-term influence. But, *Modest_Witness@Second_Millennium* shows, these foods and food-crops represent a new age, an age with many other embodiments, from 'databases' to universities, from custom-built rats to biological computer chips. Yes, it is the age of 'hypercapitalism', the time when, as the social theorist Anthony Giddens puts it, we feel ourselves living in 'a runaway world'.[23] But there is also immense creativity at work. Sometimes, this sounds like mere political cliché-mongering – Cool Britannia and all that nonsense. But Haraway shows that there is something more genuinely liberating going on. And, on the other side, there are some sinister aspects to the recoil from poor old flounderised tomatoes.

Haraway isn't trying to persuade us to buy genetic. Actually, the book leaves us to our own uncertainties as consumers. But she is warning us not to settle for some of the anti-genetic rhetoric, and also to acknowledge to ourselves the degree to which our world is changing. We need to re-tool *all* our reasons, for and against weird new foods, and for and against all kinds of other beings and concepts. At the heart of *Modest_Witness*, there is a vision of 'the time'. It is that vision which I now wish to explore, as we move towards Haraway's anti-conclusion, her refusal to settle into a fixed response or verdict.

Throughout *Modest_Witness*, one of the organising concepts is the 'chronotope': the phenomenon which represents its time. Literally, a 'chronotope' defines what is 'topical' in a period. These are the images and ideas, the objects and events in which the age finds its meanings. For Haraway, the central chronotopes of the present age are 'the gene and the computer'.[24] They are more than mere symbols, these presences – they are the means by which we organise our sense of ourselves in history. The gene and the computer are our ways of defining what makes our time different from those that went before. It is, of course, quite right to have mixed reactions to the computer and all of its associated phenomena. Haraway isn't saying that just because something is a chronotope, we have to worship it, or even like it. But it would be a mistake to think you can just get it out of your life.

One way to tell whether something is a chronotope is to try to have no view of it at all. If it really is one of the time's defining topics, you will probably find that you have a surplus of views about it, some hostile, some welcoming. Even trying to ignore the gene and the computer becomes an expression of a fundamental attitude. What you think about the gene is more than just another of your ideas and values. These are core values; they have consequences everywhere else in your life. You can easily see why the computer is a defining subject. Just remember all that anxiety about the millennium bug, how many aspects of everyday life suddenly seemed hooked up to the computer. The gene is also diffused through everyday life – after Flavr Savr, all food really *is* 'genetic food', modified or apparently unmodified. The gene stands for *your* chances of getting diseases, and gene therapy for *your* hope of avoiding them. The gene is the secret language of life chances. In our reactions to genetic foods, we are starting to explore our hopes and fears for the whole genetic age.

When genes first became a moral issue, they were all about purity: how good are your genes, how pure is your pedigree? Now the gene is all about crossing-over. What plutonium did for the elements, transgenic organisms will do for the organic realm, the species. Both the transuranic elements and the transgenic organisms are

Earthshaking artificial productions . . . whose status as aliens on earth, and indeed in the entire solar system, has changed who we are fundamentally and permanently . . . [25]

There is a famous poem by the American poet Wallace Stevens, called 'Anecdote of a Jar', in which an entire landscape folds itself around one small man-made object. For Haraway, the equivalent poem would be 'Anecdote of a Gene', say the flounder gene in one tomato or the bacterial gene in its fellow. In the Stevens poem, a vast panorama of mountains comes into new form in the presence of the jar. In Haraway's poem, the panorama of the solar system itself takes a new shape in the presence of these 'trans' genes.

How can the migratory gene be so significant? In the presence of these mobile genes, we can no longer talk with confidence about 'nature' or 'culture'. When an article claims that a modified vegetable will 'naturally' resist disease, that is a small sign that the category of 'nature' no longer exists. It has been replaced by a hybrid for which as yet there is no new name. But 'nature' and 'culture' are not just any old categories: they are connected to almost all of the big ideas through which we define and evaluate ourselves and our lives. We think of our own characteristics as partly given by nature, and partly acquired through participation in culture. Huge debates have raged, over the last four hundred years, over how far 'nature' makes us what we are, how far we are products of 'nurture'. You can see these arguments arising in Shakespeare, and you can find their direct descendants in current dilemmas about education and social policy. But every time we look at the world, we use the concepts of nature and culture to orient our gaze. That over there is a natural object – the sky, say, or those clouds. On the horizon, those shapes are man-made – the line of rooftops or the flag flying. We have become adept at scanning the world for nature and culture, and we negotiate all kinds of ambiguities with every glance. That flower bed is cultivated nature. But we also look at actions as natural or cultural. It is natural, say, to want a home; it is cultural to want plaster ducks on the wall. No more: after the migration of the gene, we are going to have to begin to unlearn these habits, if Haraway is right.

In fact, she believes that for a long time the division has been illusory. But now the illusion is being shattered by a cascade of new objects under our noses, and in our mouths: 'Potent categories collapse into each other.'[26] In Haraway's view, Western culture is in a moment of really profound transfiguration. This is the meaning that she reads into her encounter with the monster tomatoes and other genetically new beings.

All cultures depend upon categories. They are ways of dividing up the world, and indeed we have no chance to construct a world at all without these divisions, for we would be facing only a flux of shadows. Recent work in anthropology, such as George Lakoff's *Women, Fire and Dangerous Things*, has explored the central role of categories in the formation of cultures: nature and culture, fire and water, earth and air, body and spirit, male and female, all play their part. But, as Lakoff shows, categories are never nice neat boxes; they are bundles of fizzing potential for thought and experience.[27] Haraway, as a feminist, has been concerned to analyse the failings of inherited categories, and the potential for new ones. Now, in the moment of OncoMouse and FemaleMan, she senses a change which affects all the categories in Western thought. We are leaving the era when it even seemed plausible to treat our categories, like nature and culture, male and female, as fixed and bounded entities. A category never was so clear-cut in any event. But now, at the second millennium, we are witnessing the birth of the hybrid categories. The divisions will never again even *seem* fixed. We are going to have to learn to live, think and even experience afresh.

To see just how deep the change is, we can turn from Haraway back to the birth of the category in Western thought, in Aristotle's book *The*

Categories.[28] There, in the 4th century BC, Aristotle is trying to define what it means for two things to share a 'name'. He gives as his first example an anomaly: 'For instance, while a man and a portrait can properly both be called "animals", these are equivocally named.' What he means is that the category of 'animals' is not being employed in the same way if you use it for both a living man and his portrait. By contrast, the situation is no longer equivocal when you say that 'a man and an ox are called "animals"'. Then the category is uniform and unambiguous. So the first example of a category is 'animal', and the first problem that arises is precisely on the borders where nature and culture meet and are distinguished. For Aristotle, 'animal' is the prototype category. If you can't tell what you mean by 'animal' and 'not-animal', then you don't belong to his world. But what about the gene which migrates from that giant moth to the potato? It doesn't turn the vegetable *into* an animal, true, but in Haraway's terms it collapses both categories. We have to rethink what we mean when we classify things and beings.

Aristotle gives a second example. This time he wants to explain where categories stop. His term for a category here is 'genus', used in modern biology still, and he is very much preoccupied with the biological realm:

Take the genera, for example, animal and knowledge. 'Footed', 'two-footed', 'winged', 'aquatic' are among the differentiae of animal. But none will be found to distinguish a particular species of knowledge. No species of knowledge will differ from another in being 'two-footed'.

Let us pursue the dialogue. Haraway replies on behalf of the new millennium:

. . . the organism for us is an information system of a different kind . . . [29]

This is the inner significance of the postmodern encounter between Donna Haraway and Flavr Savr or OncoMouse, and, by implication, between ourselves and mutated soybeans. We don't need to love them, or even buy them. But we need,

Haraway argues, to bear witness to their meaning, to the world that they signify, a world in which both they and we might be fellow-victims or fellow-inheritors. Knowledge and animal are now overlapping categories, and in that moment all the rest of the old 'genera' will overlap in their turn. The new millennium is transgenic.

Beyond Goodies and Baddies

Is there a moral to this postmodern encounter between Donna Haraway and genetic foods? One moral is clearly missing. You cannot go to Haraway in order to find the answer to the question: is genetic food safe or unsafe? You won't leave *Modest_Witness* newly decisive about your next shopping trip. Nor will you be clearer about your views the next time you read a news item about GM technology. You won't be more confident in your outrage against Monsanto, or more definitive about Greenpeace and their tactics. But I think it would be a good thing if Haraway's ideas were more widely known, and that they would benefit the entire discussion of genetic issues, including the food controversies.

The question of what Haraway offers is insepa-rable from the larger issue of what such thinkers are for. What do we want from our cultural theo-rists and philosophers, our science historians and political analysts? What, in other words, do we want from those thinkers who deal with social, cultural and ethical topics? Do we want them to remove ambiguities, to produce a simpler world, to make the best decisions clear? Do we want thinkers to show us whether to vote for New Labour? Do we want thinkers who will decide for us whether the Internet is good or bad for us and our children? Do you want to read ideas that will leave you more certain than before – one less dilemma, one more decision? There are plenty of candidates for such a role. The shelves are full of authoritative advice and definitive prediction. Is it not the responsibility of experts to provide answers?

Haraway has a different conception of the thinker's responsibility. Her work is certainly not neutral, and she takes sides on many questions. Yet the whole effect isn't to reduce the ambiguity of the world. Instead, we leave Haraway with a more focused sense of the real ambiguity of things, an ambiguity which will have to be part of any answers that we choose to give, any commitments we make. In Haraway's approach, ambiguity and commitment go together. That is what 'grown-up' commitment is all about: recognising the ambiguities of the world, including of one's own positions.

In another context, Haraway has been a strong admirer of the work of the French philosopher, novelist and feminist Simone de Beauvoir. I suggest that Beauvoir's book *The Ethics of Ambiguity* (1947) offers a good perspective on the value of Haraway's own thinking for us, as we turn back to the confusing world of genetic controversies. For Beauvoir, writing in the immediate aftermath of the Second World War, it would be the height of irresponsibility for a serious thinker to try to make the world seem less ambiguous. Such an approach would even, in her view, diminish the humanity of all involved:

To attain his truth, man must not attempt to dispel the ambiguity of his being, but, on the contrary, to accept the task of realising it.[30]

In *The Second Sex* (1949), Beauvoir reassessed this idiom of 'man', an enterprise that Haraway continues in her treatment of 'FemaleMan'. Meanwhile, coiled within the sentence, lies a rich concept of 'the ambiguity of . . . being'. In this approach, the task of the thinker is to help people realise the full ambiguity of their own being, and of the world to which that being bears witness. No one could accuse Beauvoir of being uncommitted: she stands as a model for the modern committed thinker. But her commitment includes this embracing of ambiguity.

In the largest perspective, I believe Haraway's approach to genetic controversy carries on Beauvoir's 'ethic of ambiguity'. Every phrase of Haraway's argument presses forward in a definite direction but with a continuing sense of ambiguity.

This implosion issuing in a wonderful bestiary of cyborgs . . .

You can feel the danger of the moment, and at the same time the excitement of a changing horizon.

There can be no new possibilities which are entirely pure, not issuing from our world. These new beings are ambiguous because we ourselves put the ambiguity into them in the first place. To evade the ambiguity of 'these genetically strange inflected proprietary beings' is to run away from your own ambiguity.[31] Like Beauvoir, Haraway seeks a grown-up commitment.

The philosopher Nietzsche called one of his late works *Beyond Good and Evil.* There he demanded that we recognise 'man's comprehensiveness and multiplicity'.[32] After Beauvoir and with Haraway, perhaps we can begin to make our own commitments in a world beyond goodies and baddies, where the issues will not take our decisions for us.

When you turn back to the continuing debate about genetic foods, I think you can see why this ethic of ambiguity could be so important. On one side, you have the goodies riding to the defence of progress:

Renowned US scientists James Watson and Norman Borlaug join more than 1,000 other scientists from around the world in endorsing the 'Declaration of Scientists in Support of Agricultural Biotechnology' . . .

Business World, 21/2/2000

And in case you missed the point, you are told just who is who: 'Norman Borlaug, who is considered the "Father of the Green Revolution" . . .'! But then on the other side, you have the goodies too, the brave and outgunned seadogs defending the English coast from an invading foreigner:

Environmental activists have ambushed a ship loaded with genetically modified soya and vowed to stay on board until the cargo was returned to the United States . . .

www.ITN.co.uk , 25/2/2000

Such heroic figures seem to offer an escape, in opposite directions, from the ambiguity of being. But to embrace ambiguity does not mean to tread a nice, clear 'third way'. In fact, there is nothing ambiguous about the rhetoric of the middle ground on genetic foods, as on other issues. Here is British Prime Minister Tony Blair trying to recognise ambiguity and be right all the way:

'The potential for good highlights why we were right not to slam the door on GM food or crops without further research. The potential for harm shows why we are right to proceed very cautiously indeed.'

www.ITN.co.uk, 27/2/2000

On one side there is rightness, and the same on the other. This is the very reverse of an ethic of ambiguity.

By contrast, Haraway offers a space where we can recognise the 'wholeness and multiplicity' of these strange new beings, a multiplicity which is, in many ways, a reflection of our own creative energies coming back to greet us. Above all, we can acknowledge our kinship with these new possibilities, either as victims or as heroes. What lies beyond the goodies and baddies, beyond the old categories? Does the idea of utopia itself survive beyond the old definitions? In the light of this postmodern encounter, I suggest that any ideal future would be one which could embrace ambiguity, rather than cure or redefine it. Haraway names such a prospect 'heterogeneous well-being', a fulfilment of ambiguity rather than an escape back into definition.[33]

Further Reading

I hope this discussion might encourage readers to make their own way into the major work in question, Donna J. Haraway, *Modest_Witness@Second_Millennium. FemaleMan©_Meets_OncoMouse™*, (New York and London: Routledge, 1997). The central section for the current topic is Part II.2, 'FemaleMan©_Meets_OncoMouse™'. This covers the cyborg, transgenetic organisms, FemaleMan and OncoMouse, all from the perspective of border-crossings and ambiguities. The richest linkages then run forward to Part III.6, 'Race: Universal Donors in a Vampire Culture' (pp. 213–66), where the full moral and political consequences of the argument are unfolded.

Haraway's thinking always generates fertile interconnections. From *Modest_Witness*, these reach back most richly to her collection entitled *Simians, Cyborgs and Women* (London: Free Association Books, 1991), where the reader can find one version of the famous essay on cyborgs, under the title 'A Cyborg Manifesto: Science, Technology and Socialist-Feminism in the Late Twentieth Century'. This can also be found in Linda J. Nicholson (ed.), *Feminism/Postmodernism* (New York and London: Routledge, 1990), as 'A Manifesto For Cyborgs'. The first version appeared in *Socialist Review*, 15.80 (1985). There is a rich array of responses and dialogues in Chris Hables Gray (ed.), *The Cyborg Handbook* (New York and

London: Routledge, 1995), from which N. Katherine Hayles, 'The Life Cycle of Cyborgs' is especially relevant. Haraway's own *Cyborg Babies* (New York and London: Routledge, 1998) follows the question of technoscience into a different moral terrain.

Finally, *Modest_Witness* belongs with a group of distinguished works which have attempted to comprehend the new relationships between science, technology and culture. The most relevant are:

Ulrich Beck, *World Risk Society* (Cambridge: Polity Press, 1999).

Manuel Castells, *End of Millennium* (Malden, Mass. and Oxford: Blackwell, 1997).

Bruno Latour, *Pandora's Hope* (Cambridge, Mass. and London: Harvard University Press, 1999).

Notes

1. Haraway's most famous single work is 'A Cyborg Manifesto', originally published in 1985 and variously reprinted, including in her own collection, *Simians, Cyborgs and Women* (London: Free Association Books, 1991). Here she takes a feminist leap into the realm of science fiction futures. Additional information on Haraway's works is given in the section on Further Reading.

2. Donna J. Haraway, *Modest_Witness@Second_Millennium. Female Man©_ Meets_OncoMouse™* (New York and London: Routledge, 1997), p. 62.

3. Ibid., p. 88.

4. The genes of this tomato and its suspect kin are identified on pp. 59–60 of *Modest_Witness*.

5. The transuranic elements and the new genetics are set in context on pp. 51–6 of *Modest_Witness*.

6. Ibid., p. 85.

7. Ibid., p. 57.

8. Ibid., p. 60, where Haraway makes her confession of style.

9. Ibid., pp. 88–9, on the revolution in kinship.

10. Haraway's declaration on behalf of her cyborgs is made on p. 12 of *Modest_Witness*, except for the definition of Machine and Human, from p. 59.

11. The vivid response to the appearance of Onco-

Mouse™ is given on p. 79 of *Modest_Witness*, except for the definition of Machine and Human, from p. 59.

12. The treatment of hypercapital and the globe appears on pp. 12–14 of *Modest_Witness*.

13. Ibid., p. 54.

14. The impassioned critique of racist reverberation is carried forward on pp. 60–2 of *Modest_Witness*.

15. The theme of purity echoes across *Modest_Witness*, as these quotes show. Purity Hall is identified on p. 86, the alien genes are from p. 62, and the idea of a genetic re-mix is on p. 121.

16. The history and critique of 'modest witnessing' is on pp. 22–4 of *Modest_Witness*.

17. Ibid., p. 8.

18. The discussion of perspective evolves through *Modest_Witness* from p. 52 on the rodent viewpoint, to p. 70 on FemaleMan and p. 84 on narrative itself. The twisting form of this discussion helps to convey the essential idea.

19. Ibid., p. 121.

20. Ibid., p. 80.

21. The analysis of the new research institutes is carried out on pp. 90–7 of *Modest_Witness*.

22. The analysis of worlds and their knowledge is on p. 37 of *Modest_Witness*.

23. Anthony Giddens, *The Runaway World* (London: Profile, 1999).

24. The 'chronotope' is introduced on pp. 41–2 of *Modest_Witness*.

25. Ibid., p. 55.

26. Ibid., p. 68.

27. George Lakoff, *Women, Fire and Dangerous Things: What Categories Reveal About The Mind* (Chicago. University of Chicago Press, 1987).

28. Aristotle, *The Categories*, translated by H. P. Cooke (Cambridge, Mass.: Harvard University Press, 1938). The examples are taken from Book I.

29. *Modest_Witness*, p. 97.

30. Simone de Beauvoir, *The Ethics of Ambiguity*, translated by B. Frechtman (New York: Capitol Press, 1996), p. 13.

31. The vision of the imploding bestiary is on p. 43 of *Modest_Witness*.

32. The quotation is from the translation in *The Portable Nietzsche*, edited and translated by W. Kaufmann (New York: Penguin, 1954), p. 445.

33. The assertion of a new well-being is made on p. 95 of *Modest_Witness*.